T0000741

ESCAPING WARS AND WAVES

ENCOUNTERS WITH SYRIAN REFUGEES

HEADING TOWARDS DOVER

P&O

Pride of Burgundy
DOVER

DRAWN & RECORDED BY OLIVIER KUGLER

GRAPHIC MUNDI

"BY NOW,
ALL THE SURVIVORS, ALL WHO AVOIDED HEADLONG DEATH
WERE SAFE AT HOME, ESCAPED THE WARS AND WAVES."

FROM THE ODYSSEY BY HOMER, TRANSLATION © ROBERT FAGLES, 1996

CATALOGING-IN-PUBLICATION DATA IS ON FILE WITH THE LIBRARY OF CONGRESS.

FIRST PUBLISHED BY EDITION MODERNE AS DEM KRIEG ENTRONNEN
COPYRIGHT © 2017 EDITION MODERNE, ZURICH, SWITZERLAND, AND OLIVIER KUGLER
ALL RIGHTS RESERVED.
THIS EDITION COPYRIGHT © OLIVIER KUGLER 2023
PUBLISHED BY THE PENNSYLVANIA STATE UNIVERSITY PRESS,
UNIVERSITY PARK, PA 16802-1003
FIRST PUBLISHED IN ENGLISH BY MYRIAD EDITIONS, WWW.MYRIADEDITIONS.COM

10 9 8 7 6 5 4 3 2 1

graphic mundi
drawing our worlds together

GRAPHIC MUNDI IS AN IMPRINT OF THE PENNSYLVANIA STATE UNIVERSITY PRESS.

THE PENNSYLVANIA STATE UNIVERSITY PRESS IS A MEMBER OF THE ASSOCIATION OF
UNIVERSITY PRESSES.

IT IS THE POLICY OF THE PENNSYLVANIA STATE UNIVERSITY PRESS TO USE ACID-FREE PAPER.
PUBLICATIONS ON UNCOATED STOCK SATISFY THE MINIMUM REQUIREMENTS OF AMERICAN
NATIONAL STANDARD FOR INFORMATION SCIENCES- PERMANENCE OF PAPER FOR PRINTED
LIBRARY MATERIAL, ANSI Z 39.48-1992.

Supported using public funding by
**ARTS COUNCIL
ENGLAND**
LOTTERY FUNDED

"**HELLO**, MY NAME IS OLIVIER KUGLER, I AM A GERMAN REPORTAGE ILLUSTRATOR BASED IN LONDON. MÉDECINS SANS FRONTIÈRES COMMISSIONED ME TO PORTRAY SYRIAN REFUGEES, IN ORDER TO HELP RAISE AWARENESS ABOUT THEIR SITUATION. MAY I INTERVIEW AND TAKE PHOTOS OF YOU? THE PHOTOS WON'T BE PUBLISHED, BUT I NEED THEM AS REFERENCE FOR MY DRAWINGS." These were the words I used to introduce myself to Syrian refugees I met in Iraqi Kurdistan, Greece and France. Based on these encounters, which took place between 2013 and 2017, I created the drawings and texts which are collected in this book.

In December 2013 I travelled together with Julien Rey from Médecins sans Frontières (MSF) to Domiz Refugee camp. Accompanied by two Syrian Kurds, Mazen and Amer, who helped us with translations, we met open-hearted people who invited us into their tents and houses where they told us over a cup of tea about their lives back home, their escape from Syria and about the living conditions in the camp. Not all of the people I interviewed, or wanted to interview, were happy about the idea that their portraits would be published. Some were afraid that their relatives back in Syria, or they themselves, could get into trouble with one of the many warring factions in the conflict... or even with the authorities in the camp. There were also problems with my attempts to interview and photograph women. I would have loved to have depicted the busy goings-on inside one of the camp's beauty parlors, the young women putting on makeup and getting their hair done ahead of a wedding party, or the chain-smoking old lady who worked as a midwife... unfortunately, all my requests were turned down.

In the beginning of July 2015, I was asked by MSF if I would like to visit the Greek island of Kos to report on the stranded refugees. During my stay there, I frequently cycled out to the beaches, where, in the early morning, people arrived in overcrowded rubber dinghies. After they got themselves registered, they were told that they weren't allowed to board the next ferry to Athens. Instead they would have to wait, sometimes for weeks, for the documents that would give them permission to continue their journeys to Northern Europe. The local authorities provided neither accommodation nor showers or toilets for the refugees; many of them were sent to a dilapidated and already over-crowded hotel on the outskirts of the town, where a small MSF team looked after them. Other than in Domiz I found it relatively easy to get permission from women to take their pictures while they told me their stories. Nevertheless, I noticed that they weren't very comfortable with it – who would want to be photographed by a complete stranger in such a situation? But it was important to me that their voices should be heard, that they could share their stories, their frustration and their anger over the lack of support from the Greek authorities. One lady told me:

"IN EUROPE, I HAD HOPED, WE WOULD GET TREATED WITH RESPECT."

In 2016, during the Easter holidays, I took the ferry to Calais where I spent three days in the migrant camp, known as 'The Jungle.' Compared to Domiz and Kos, I found it even more difficult to meet people who were happy with me interviewing and photographing them. The camp at this time, was in the focus of the media. Perhaps many of the refugees became irritated with all the cameras being constantly pointed at them. Luckily, a member of the local MSF team helped me talk with some of the camp's residents.

In London, my studio is located in the same building as the Woman's Refugee Association. I told them about my work and they introduced me to Dr. Wafaa from Damascus, who attended their English language lessons.

Counterpoints Arts, an organization that supports art projects made by and about refugees, helped me to get a grant from the Arts Council England, which allowed me to work on this book. It was in the Counterpoints Arts office that I spotted the photo of a smiling boy with dark curly hair. It was Mohamad: he and his family had found refuge in Birmingham, where I visited them in October 2016.

Just after Christmas 2016, I spent some days at my parents' house. They introduced me to a family who had to leave their home in Deir-ez-Zor, Syria, and – for the time being – are now living in Simmozheim, in the Black Forest, the village where I grew up.

I am very grateful that I had the chance to meet the people I portrayed in my drawings. I feel connected to them and want to thank them very much for their patience and trust. I hope that their circumstances have improved significantly and wish them, and their compatriots, all the best!

KURDISTAN REGION

(IRAQ)

THE CAMP'S GATE

DON'T TAKE PHOTOS CLOSE TO THE CAMP'S ENTRANCE!
YOU WILL GET IN TROUBLE WITH THE PESHMERGA GUARDING THE CAMP.

MILITARY FORCES OF THE AUTONOMOUS
REGION OF IRAQI KURDISTAN.

WATER OR SEWAGE TANKER?

AUTHOR'S NOTE:

I met Muhamed one cold and wet morning in front
of the guarded entrance to the camp where I was
waiting for my translator (who was late) to arrive.
The vendor must have seen me standing there shivering,
forlorn... and brought me a steaming cup of sweet
instant coffee that tasted surprisingly good. When
I wanted to pay for the coffee he repeatedly refused
my payment.

MUHAMED'S TEA CART

PARASOL

STANDING ON BROKEN CINDER BLOCKS TO KEEP HIS FEET OUT OF THE MUD.

TAXI

"WE FLED SYRIA FIFTEEN MONTHS AGO.

WE HAD BEEN LIVING IN DAMASCUS FOR MANY YEARS. ONE AFTERNOON WE COULD HEAR A HELICOPTER APPROACHING. IT RANDOMLY STARTED BOMBING HOUSES IN OUR NEIGHBORHOOD. WE RAN AWAY FROM OUR HOUSE JUST IN TIME — IT WAS HIT BY A BOMB AND DESTROYED. IT WAS NOT SAFE TO STAY... AS I'VE GOT SEVEN DAUGHTERS I WAS VERY WORRIED THAT THEY WOULD GET RAPED... WE LEFT DAMASCUS IMMEDIATELY BY BUS WITH NOTHING BUT THE CLOTHES WE'D BEEN WEARING. THE JOURNEY TO QUAMISHLI WAS SCARY AS THERE ARE MANY CHECKPOINTS. THEY ARE MANNED BY EITHER THE SYRIAN ARMY, THE FREE SYRIAN ARMY, OR JIHADIST GROUPS. BUT WE MADE IT AND WERE ABLE TO STAY FOR A WHILE WITH MY FATHER-IN-LAW'S FAMILY. BUT I HAVE A LARGE FAMILY, SO WE COULDN'T STAY WITH THEM FOR LONG. BECAUSE OF THE WAR THERE IS NO WORK IN THE AREA. FOOD, ELECTRICITY, AND FUEL ARE SCARCE AND EXPENSIVE SO WE LEFT FOR IRAQI KURDISTAN. NOW, IN THE CAMP, WE ALL LIVE IN ONE TENT. I AM HAPPY THAT WE ARE ALL TOGETHER BUT I AM NOT HAPPY WITH THE LIVING CONDITIONS HERE... THE RAIN, THE COLD... THERE IS WATER EVERYWHERE. I HAVE A BIG FAMILY TO LOOK AFTER BUT I AM OLD AND I AM SICK..."

CRIES WHEN HE STARTS TALKING ABOUT HIS WIFE:

IT HAD JUST STARTED TO SNOW

✳ THE PLAYGROUND

BECAUSE THE CAMP SOON BECAME OVERCROWDED, NEW ARRIVALS PITCHED THEIR TENTS IN FRONT OF THE FENCE SECURING THE CAMP'S SOUTHEASTERN BORDER. THIS AREA WAS ORIGINALLY EARMARKED BY THE PLANNERS TO SERVE AS A RECREATIONAL AREA THAT WOULD HAVE INCLUDED A FOOTBALL PITCH AND A PLAYGROUND.

AUTHOR'S NOTE:

Julien, Mazen (our translator) and I had spent the best part of an hour in the family's tent when I noticed some movement underneath the blankets on top of the matress: ⟶

one of Ahmed's teenage sons had been hiding there... Was he embarrassed?
I didn't want to ask.

"**WE'VE** BEEN LIVING HERE IN DOMIZ FOR ABOUT ONE AND A HALF YEARS. LAST YEAR MY BROTHER-IN-LAW AND I BOUGHT SOME BUILDING MATERIALS AND STARTED TO BUILD US A SMALL LITTLE HOUSE AND THIS WORK SHOP. IT IS NOT FINISHED YET BUT IT SHOULD GET US THROUGH THE WINTER.

".**I**'VE ALWAYS BEEN FASCINATED BY ELECTRICAL APPLIANCES. WHEN EVER MY PARENTS BOUGHT A NEW RECORD PLAYER OR RADIO IT DIDN'T TAKE LONG UNTIL I GOT MY HANDS ON IT AND EVENTUALLY BROKE IT. **WHEN** I WAS ABOUT TEN YEARS OLD I STARTED TO VISIT THE WORKSHOP RUN BY A FRIEND OF MY FATHER. HE TAUGHT ME HOW TO REPAIR ELECTRICAL APPLIANCES. THIS BECAME MY HOBBY AND LATER MY JOB.

"**I** WANT TO TRAVEL TO EUROPE. AS I DON'T HAVE A PASSPORT I CAN'T DO IT LEGALLY. FIFTEEN YEARS AGO I PAID A TRAFFICKER 5,000 US DOLLARS TO TAKE ME TO CYPRUS AND FROM THERE ON TO ITALY... IT TURNED OUT HE WAS A CHEAT AND RAN AWAY WITH THE MONEY. I TRIED IT AGAIN A COUPLE MORE TIMES BUT NO LUCK! AFTERWARDS I GOT MARRIED AND HAD CHILDREN."

A CUSTOMER AND HIS SON PICKING UP A REPAIRED TV SET

PORTRAIT OF A WOMAN DRAWN ON THE WALL

"**ONE** OF MY OTHER PASSIONS IS MUSIC. IN DAMASCUS I ALSO USED TO WORK AS A MUSICIAN. MY SIBLINGS AND I USED TO EARN GOOD MONEY PLAYING AT WEDDINGS AND OTHER PARTIES. I ESPECIALLY ENJOYED PLAYING THE TAMBOUR. ✳ I ALSO USED TO PERFORM IN A CASINO. THERE, THOUGH WE HAD TO PLAY ARABIC MUSIC AS OUR KURDISH MUSIC WAS NOT WELCOMED.

"**WHEN** THE WAR STARTED I DIDN'T SEE ANY FUTURE FOR MY FAMILY IN OUR COUNTRY. AGAIN, WE DECIDED TO GO TO EUROPE. I PAID A TRAFFICKER TO TAKE US TO TURKEY AND FROM THERE TO GREECE... IT TURNED OUT, AGAIN, THAT THE GUY WAS A FRAUD. WITH NO SAVINGS LEFT, WE HAD TO SELL MY WIFE'S JEWELLERY IN ORDER TO FLEE TO KURDISTAN. IRAQI ↗

✳ KURDISH TRADITIONAL INSTRUMENT... → A LONG NECKED LUTE.

"**WE** ARE FORTUNATE IN BEING WELCOMED BY OUR BROTHERS IN KURDISTAN BUT I DON'T SEE ANY FUTURE FOR US HERE EITHER. I DON'T PLAY MUSIC ANYMORE AS I DON'T FEEL HAPPY. INSTEAD I WORK HERE IN MY SHOP. THERE IS A LOT OF DEMAND AND MY WORK IS WELL RESPECTED. I USUALLY WORK UNTIL MIDNIGHT... I WANT TO SAVE MONEY... BUT I ALSO REPAIR APPLIANCES FOR FREE IF THE CUSTOMER HAS GOT NO MONEY.

"**A** COUSIN OF MINE LIVES IN BULGARIA WHERE HE IS DOING QUITE WELL. HE TOLD ME IT IS RELATIVELY EASY AND SAFE TO GET THERE. MAYBE NEXT YEAR OR THE YEAR AFTER WE WILL GO TO EUROPE, INSHALLAH."

DJWAN'S SOUND SYSTEM RENTAL

THE BUSINESS IS GOING OK …

TWO ARMCHAIRS COVERED WITH A BLANKET

GIRL DANCING (THE MUSIC HASN'T STARTED YET)

"**I RENT** OUT THE SYSTEM ABOUT TWICE A WEEK, WHEN THERE IS A WEDDING, A BIRTHDAY PARTY OR WHEN A BABY IS BORN.

"**WE** GET BETWEEN 75,000 IQD* AND 100,000 IQD (51 GBP) FOR EACH RENTAL.

*IRAQI DINAR

"**I** DON'T OWN THE BUSINESS… SETTING IT UP THOUGH WAS MY IDEA. AS I DIDN'T HAVE ANY MONEY A FRIEND OF MINE BOUGHT THE EQUIPMENT ABOUT A MONTH AGO FOR ABOUT 3,500 US DOLLARS AND THEN EMPLOYED ME TO RENT IT OUT AND TO OPERATE IT.

"**I** HAVE ALWAYS BEEN INTERESTED IN MUSIC. I COME FROM AN ARTISTIC FAMILY. HMMM… OK, MY FATHER AND MOTHER LIKE ART… OR AT LEAST THEY DON'T DISLIKE IT. MY BROTHERS AND I, OUR WHOLE FAMILY, WE USED TO SING A LOT WHEN WE WERE YOUNGER. NONE OF US WAS ANY GOOD AT SINGING BUT WE REALLY LOVED DOING IT!

"**I** DO LIKE ALL KINDS OF MUSIC BUT MY FAVOURITE SINGER IS MUHAMMAD SHEKHO, A VERY POPULAR SINGER FROM QUAMISHLI WHERE I GREW UP."

"THE TRADITION WANTS IT THAT THE BRIDE SITS ON THE LEFT HAND SIDE AND THE GROOM ON THE RIGHT HAND SIDE."

AUTHOR'S NOTE:
One late afternoon at the camp's north-western perimeter, we met a young man setting up a sound system for a wedding celebration. We were only able to have a brief chat with him as we had to leave soon (MSF employees are required to leave the camp before night fall).

Djwan invited us to visit him in his shop.

PREPARING TEA →

GENEROUS WITH THE SUGAR!

PLASTIC LEAVES

HOW DID I FEEL ABOUT BEING A SOLDIER IN THE GOVERNMENT ARMY?

ARE YOU KIDDING?

OF COURSE I AM NOT A SUPPORTER OF AL-ASSAD.

→ I HAD TO DO MY MILITARY SERVICE BECAUSE IT WAS MANDATORY.

"**I WAS ONE** YEAR INTO MY MILITARY SERVICE WHEN THE PROTESTS KICKED OFF IN 2011... A LITTLE LATER THE WAR STARTED.

"**AT** THE BEGINNING I THOUGHT THAT EVERYTHING WOULD BE OVER SOON. BUT DAY AFTER DAY IT BECAME OBVIOUS THAT THE SITUATION WOULD ONLY BECOME WORSE.

"**MY** DETACHMENT WAS BASED IN THE COUNTRYSIDE SURROUNDING DAMASCUS WHERE WE WERE FIGHTING THE OPPOSITION, OR THE TERRORISTS, AS OUR OFFICERS USED TO CALL THEM.

"**M**ANY OF MY FRIENDS DIED...

DURING ONE MISSION IN BOYEDAH I WAS ON THE ROOF OF A SCHOOL. I WAS SUPPOSED TO SURVEY THE AREA WHERE MY DETACHMENT WAS ADVANCING AND TAKE PRECAUTIONS IN CASE OF AN ATTACK. THE ADVANCE WAS HEADED BY A TANK. A MAN IN DISGUISE APPROACHED AND MANAGED TO SHOOT OUR COLONEL. WHILE THIS WAS HAPPENING I TRIED TO SHOOT THE ATTACKER WITH MY SNIPER RIFLE AND I WAS CALLING AND SCREAMING AT MY COMRADES FOR HELP.

"MOMENTS LATER A ROCKET-PROPELLED GRENADE WAS LAUNCHED AND HIT THE TANK DEAD ON. THERE WAS A LOT OF FIRE... TWO OF MY FRIENDS WERE IN THE TANK. **THEY BURNED TO DEATH...** THEY BECAME ASHES.

SEVEN OF US WERE KILLED IN THIS ATTACK..."

MEDECINS SANS FR

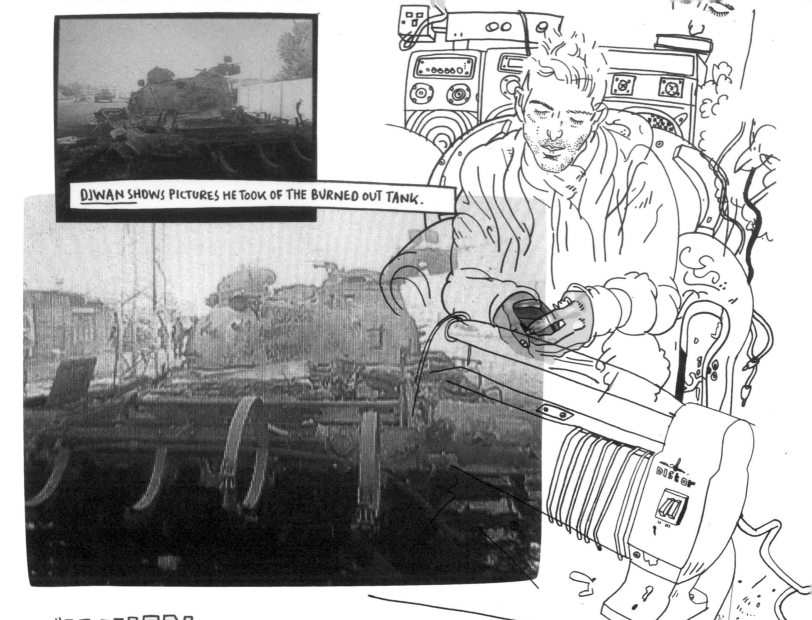

DJWAN SHOWS PICTURES HE TOOK OF THE BURNED OUT TANK.

"**WHEN** I WAS A CHILD I ALWAYS WANTED TO BECOME A TEACHER... THIS WAS MY DREAM. IT DIDN'T MATTER TO ME WHAT KIND OF TEACHER... JUST BECOMING ANY KIND OF TEACHER SEEMED TO BE FINE TO ME. WHEN I WAS 16 I STARTED HELPING OUT IN MY UNCLE'S BUTCHER SHOP, WHEN I CAME BACK FROM HIGH SCHOOL IN THE AFTERNOON. I HATED IT BECAUSE OF THE ANIMALS' BLOOD. IT WAS DISGUSTING! I WORKED THERE UNTIL I WENT TO LEBANON.

"I WAS 19 WHEN I WENT TO JONIEH, LEBANON, TO WORK THERE AS A WAITER IN A BAR. I WENT THERE LIKE EVERYBODY ELSE, TO SAVE SOME MONEY IN ORDER TO GET ME THROUGH MY MILITARY SERVICE. BECAUSE YOU WILL DIE OF HUNGER IF YOU RELY ON THE ARMY LOOKING AFTER YOU. (DJWAN LAUGHS A LOT AFTER HE SAYS THIS.) I DIDN'T HAVE A GOOD TIME IN JONIEH. EVEN THOUGH THE TOWN IS A BEAUTIFUL AND POPULAR MEDITERRANEAN RESORT... I HAD TO WORK LONG HOURS. IT WAS EXHAUSTING AND I COULD HARDLY FIND THE TIME TO DO ANYTHING FUN.

"**S**EVERAL MONTHS AFTER MY ARRIVAL IN LEBANON MY FATHER PASSED AWAY. I WANTED TO GO AND SEE HIS BODY AND ATTEND THE FUNERAL BUT AS SOON AS I CROSSED THE BORDER INTO SYRIA I WAS ARRESTED BY THE MILITARY POLICE. I WAS IMMEDIATELY DRAFTED INTO THE ARMY AND WASN'T ABLE TO SEE MY FATHER'S BODY...

"WE HAVE TO START OUR MILITARY SERVICE AT THE AGE OF 18... I JOINED LATE. WHEN YOU SHOW UP LATE THE MILITARY POLICE WILL DEFINITELY CAPTURE YOU AS EVERYBODY KNOWS... EVEN IF YOU ARE HIDING ON THE MOON!"

"BEFORE EVERY NEW MISSION OUR COMMANDING OFFICER TOLD US: 'EVERYTHING IS FINE. DON'T BE SCARED. YOU ARE HERE TO FIGHT FOR YOUR PEOPLE.'

WAS I SCARED?

NO ONE CAN SAY: 'I AM A MAN AND THEREFORE I AM NOT AFRAID.' WE WERE ALL SCARED. YOU HOPE TO SURVIVE ONE MISSION. WHEN THE MISSION IS OVER ANOTHER ONE COMES AND YOU ARE AWARE THAT YOU COULD GET KILLED AT ANY GIVEN MOMENT.

"HOW DID I BECOME A SNIPER? I BECAME A SNIPER BY DRAWING LOTS... AT THE BEGINNING OF MILITARY SERVICE THEY USUALLY DECIDE WHAT EACH RECRUIT WILL DO AT RANDOM.

WHAT I LIKED ABOUT THE ARMY WAS THE CAMARADERIE... I MADE VERY GOOD FRIENDS.

"ONE OF MY FRIENDS SHOT HIMSELF WITH HIS RIFLE. THREE BULLETS... TWO OF THEM PENETRATED HIS BODY AND THE THIRD ONE WENT INTO THE AIR. MY COMMANDER PUT ME IN JAIL BECAUSE OF THAT. WE USED TO LIVE IN THE SAME TENT AND THE COMMANDER ACCUSED ME OF KILLING MY FRIEND.

"I DON'T KNOW WHY HE KILLED HIMSELF EXACTLY... IT MUST HAVE BEEN AN ACCUMULATION OF EVENTS. HIS FATHER HAD ALREADY BEEN DEAD FOR A LONG TIME AND HIS MOTHER HAD DIED RECENTLY... THE COMMANDER DID NOT LET HIM ATTEND HER FUNERAL. ON TOP OF THAT HIS BROTHER WAS MURDERED. SINCE THEN HIS SISTER HAD BEEN SUFFERING FROM DEPRESSION. A COUPLE OF DAYS BEFORE MY FRIEND KILLED HIMSELF HE RECEIVED A PHONE CALL FROM HIS UNCLE WHO TOLD HIM THAT HIS SISTER HAD GONE OUT INTO THE STREET AND STARTED SCREAMING UNCONTROLLABLY... THAT SHE HAD BECOME COMPLETELY CRAZY.

"SO MY COMMANDING OFFICERS STARTED AN INVESTIGATION INCLUDING A LOT OF INTERROGATION AND TORTURE. THEY HUNG ME FROM THE PRISON'S CEILING AND BEAT ME. THEY WHIP YOU AND ELECTROCUTE YOU UNTIL YOU CONFESS TO SOMETHING YOU DIDN'T DO. THEY ALSO KEPT ON INSULTING ME AND SAID TERRIBLE THINGS ABOUT MEMBERS OF MY FAMILY. OF COURSE THE FOOD WAS DISGUSTING AND THE PORTIONS WERE SMALL. I WAS ALWAYS HUNGRY. AFTER A WEEK THEY REALIZED I HAD NOT KILLED MY FRIEND.

"WHEN I ARRIVED IN DOMIZ I FELT VERY SAD... I WAS ALLOCATED A SPACE IN A TENT WITH FIVE OTHER GUYS. THE TENT IS LOCATED IN THE CAMP'S SINGLE MEN'S AREA. THE LIVING CONDITIONS THERE ARE BAD. THERE IS ALWAYS A SHORTAGE OF WATER... WE HAVE THE FEELING THAT WE ARE BEING NEGLECTED BY EVERYONE."

SOME OF MY FRIENDS WHO NOTED MY DEPRESSION ENCOURAGED ME TO SEE NIHAD

THE MSF MENTAL HEALTH WORKER WHO VISITS THE SINGLE MEN'S AREA FROM TIME TO TIME.

THANK GOD I MET NIHAD.

I HAVE ALWAYS FELT VERY MUCH AT EASE WHEN I TALK WITH HIM.

SOMETIMES I HAVE NIGHTMARES.

I AM A TEACHER NOW.

I TEACH BREAKDANCING AND RAPPING TO 9-16 YEAR OLDS.

HERE ARE SOME OF MY STUDENTS.

DURING THEIR LUNCH BREAK ON THEIR WAY HOME FROM SCHOOL, THEY OFTEN COME BY MY PLACE TO SAY HELLO.

HELLO!

GRINS LIKE A CHESHIRE CAT

DJWAN (HAPPY!) ☺
TAKING PICTURES ON HIS MOBILE

UNHCR

"WHEN I WAS A KID I DID A LITTLE BIT OF BREAKDANCING WITH MY OLDER BROTHERS. IN MY SPARE TIME IN LEBANON I TOOK CLASSES IN BREAKDANCING AND PRACTISED WHENEVER I HAD THE CHANCE.

"AFTER I ARRIVED IN DOMIZ I THOUGHT IT WOULD BE NICE TO TEACH THE KIDS.

"I SUGGESTED MY IDEA TO THE IRC ✳ AND THEY ACCEPTED IT... SO THEY PROVIDED US WITH A TENT TO PRACTISE IN.
✳ INTERNATIONAL RESCUE COMMITTEE

"WORKING WITH THE KIDS MAKES ME FEEL MORE THAN HAPPY. I FEEL PROUD OF MYSELF WHENEVER I TEACH THEM. IT'S GREAT!

"THE SITUATION BACK IN QUAMISHLI IS BAD AND THE PEOPLE OVER THERE DON'T SEE THE SITUATION GETTING ANY BETTER SOON. I THINK A LOT OF PEOPLE WOULD LOVE TO COME OVER TO IRAQI KURDISTAN. BUT SINCE THE BORDER HAS BEEN CLOSED IT HAS BECOME DIFFICULT FOR PEOPLE TO MAKE THE CROSSING."

GREECE

REZAN,
FASHION DESIGNER

"**ABOUT** TWO YEARS AGO WE WERE WAITING FOR THE ISLAMIC STATE TO ENTER OUR CITY. FROM THIS POINT ON OUR LIVES BECAME REALLY DIFFICULT. IT STARTED WITH THINGS BECOMING VERY EXPENSIVE. WHEN THE ISLAMIC STATE ENTERED OUR CITY, WE AND AROUND 200,000 OTHER PEOPLE FLED TO THE TURKISH BORDER. AT THE BEGINNING, TURKISH AUTHORITIES PREVENTED US FROM ENTERING THEIR COUNTRY. FINALLY THEY OPENED THE BORDER FOR US."

WE ARE A GROUP OF 16 PEOPLE FROM KOBANI. WE WANT TO GO TO GERMANY!

I CAN'T SWIM.

ROCCA, 8 YEARS OLD (NIECE OF REZAN) SHE SAYS THE BOAT JOURNEY TO KOS WAS DARK. SHE WAS VERY SCARED AND GOT SEASICK. HER UNCLE WAS HOLDING HER LIKE HE IS HOLDING HER RIGHT NOW; HE WAS HUGGING HER ALL THE TIME.

"**MOST** OF THE MEN AND SOME WOMEN WENT BACK TO KOBANI TO FREE OUR CITY. FROM OUR CAMP, ABOUT FIVE KILOMETERS AWAY FROM KOBANI, WE COULD HEAR THE FIGHTING AND SEE THE EXPLOSIONS. WE COULD ALSO HEAR THE AMERICAN FIGHTER PLANES BOMBARDING ISLAMIC STATE POSITIONS.

"**AFTER** A LONG FIGHT, OUR DEFENSE FORCES MANAGED TO CHASE THE ISLAMIC STATE OUT OF THE CITY. I WENT BACK TO CHECK ON OUR HOUSE. I DIDN'T CRY WHEN I SAW THAT OUR HOUSE HAD BEEN RANSACKED. I WAS VERY HAPPY THAT MY IMMEDIATE FAMILY WAS ALIVE. IT WAS WHEN I SAW THE TREES THAT I COULDN'T HOLD BACK—THE ISLAMIC STATE HAD BLOWN UP ALL THE TREES IN AN ORCHARD THAT BELONGED TO OUR NEXT-DOOR NEIGHBOR. I USED TO PLAY THERE WHEN I WAS A CHILD. I HELPED OUT DURING THE SUMMER. YOU CAN REBUILD A HOUSE EASILY, BUT THE TREES? IT TOOK A LOT OF TIME AND CARE FOR THEM TO GROW AND PROSPER."

"ART SUPPLIES AMID THE RUBBLE OF MY STUDIO: I TOOK THE WATER COLORS WITH ME. THEY ARE HERE IN MY BACKPACK. I USED TO HAVE A LOT OF MY ARTWORK HANGING ON THE WALLS. THE ISLAMIC STATE DESTROYED IT ALL."

DESTROYED BUILDING: "THIS IS WHAT IS LEFT OF THE SCHOOL WHERE I USED TO GIVE PAINTING LESSONS. IT GOT HIT BY AN AMERICAN WARPLANE."

OMAR
MEDICAL STUDENT

① "IN SYRIA THERE WAS A TIME WHEN I WASN'T THINKING ABOUT MY FUTURE ANYMORE; I WAS ONLY THINKING ABOUT STAYING ALIVE. FOR SIX WEEKS I SURVIVED BY EATING DISGUSTING FOOD. THE REGIME'S ARMY SURROUNDED OUR NEIGHBORHOOD (IN DOUMA, A CITY NORTHEAST OF DAMASCUS) AND DIDN'T LET ANY FOOD IN.

WE WERE EATING FOOD, MAINLY BREAD, THAT WAS RUINED, INEDIBLE, MOLDY. PEOPLE STARTED KILLING THEIR CATS TO HAVE MEAT, DONKEYS TOO.

THEY EVEN KILLED A LION IN THE ZOO TO EAT IT!

② "I VOLUNTARILY WORKED FOR THE RED CROSS/RED CRESCENT (RC/RC) BECAUSE I HAVEN'T GRADUATED YET I COULDN'T DO THE WORK OF A DOCTOR, BUT IN THE END, IN SYRIA RIGHT NOW, WHEN YOU WORK FOR THE RC/RC THEY DON'T CARE VERY MUCH ABOUT WHAT YOU ARE SPECIALIZED IN OR WHAT DEGREE YOU'VE GOT. AS LONG AS YOU HAVE KNOWLEDGE, THEY WILL TAKE YOU ON, SINCE THE NUMBER OF PEOPLE HELPING IS SO SMALL.

③ "I WAS WORKING IN THE CARS WHICH BROUGHT WOUNDED PEOPLE TO THE HOSPITAL. MANY OF THE VICTIMS LOST LIMBS IN EXPLOSIONS. OUR CARS WERE SMALL, AND THERE WERE ONLY A FEW OF THEM. SOMETIMES WE DIDN'T HAVE ENOUGH TIME AND WE COULDN'T GET ALL THE WOUNDED OUT. ESPECIALLY AFTER ONE ATTACK WITH CHEMICAL WEAPONS. THERE WERE SO MANY INJURED PEOPLE LYING AROUND DYING, WE HAD TO PRIORITIZE SAVING THE CHILDREN. THERE WAS NO OTHER SOLUTION...

⑤ "OF COURSE I MISS MY FAMILY AND MY FRIENDS. I MISS OUR HOUSE. MY BOOKS! I HAVE A LOT OF MEDICAL BOOKS. I ACTUALLY MISS THE LONG NIGHTS WHEN I DIDN'T SLEEP BECAUSE I WAS STUDYING FOR MY EXAMS. I WANT TO GO TO GERMANY. THE UNIVERSITIES THERE ARE VERY GOOD. THIS IS WHAT I REALLY CARE ABOUT. I KNOW IT WILL BE HARD TO LEARN THE LANGUAGE. IT WILL PROBABLY TAKE ME A YEAR OF INTENSE STUDYING, BUT I WILL MANAGE. I AM LOOKING FORWARD TO THIS. I JUST WANT TO FIND A SAFE PLACE AND RESTART MY LIFE, STUDY, BUILD A FAMILY."

④ A LOT OF DOCTORS FLED THE COUNTRY; THEY DIDN'T STAY TO HELP.

AS FAR AS I KNOW THERE ARE ONLY TWO DOCTORS LEFT IN THE WHOLE CITY OF DOUMA.

I HAVE A VERY BAD CONSCIENCE ABOUT LEAVING MY COUNTRY.

I DIDN'T WANT TO LEAVE;

MY FATHER ASKED ME TO...

I GAVE IN AND LEFT WITH MY BROTHER.

CATERINA

SPOT WHERE OMAR'S DINGHY LANDED

KOS ISLAND

FRANCE

③ WE TRIED TO GO TO ARABIAN COUNTRIES.

GETTING A VISA FROM THE GULF STATES IS IMPOSSIBLE.

"BUT IT IS NOT POSSIBLE AT ALL. FOR ONE AND A HALF YEARS I TRIED TO GET A VISA FOR SAUDI ARABIA. BUT IT DIDN'T LEAD ANYWHERE."

JORDAN? WE CAN'T GO TO JORDAN. THEY CLOSED THE BORDER FOR REFUGEES.

"THERE ARE ALREADY ABOUT ONE MILLION SYRIANS IN THE COUNTRY."

I CAN ONLY GO TO TURKEY.

I USED TO BE AN ENGLISH TEACHER IN SYRIA.

"WHAT WOULD I DO IN TURKEY? WORK IN A FACTORY FOR 12 HOURS A DAY TO EARN 300 US DOLLARS A MONTH? JUST TO BE ABLE TO AFFORD A ROOM I WOULD SHARE WITH THREE OTHER PEOPLE?"

THE TURKISH LANGUAGE IS VERY HARD TO LEARN ...

I COULDN'T LEARN IT.

SALT

GAS COOKER

✳ "RAZOR WIRE IS MOUNTED ON TOP OF THE FENCES. WE PUT SLEEPING BAGS OR JACKETS ON TOP TO PROTECT US. THEN WE JUMP.

"STILL, EVERY TIME I RETURN TO THE CAMP WITH CUTS ON MY HANDS AND RUINED CLOTHES."

④ AND FOR LEBANON YOU NEED TO GET A VISA NOW.

TO GET A VISA YOU NEED: A TICKET FOR A FLIGHT LEAVING BEIRUT → AND →

A HOTEL ROOM RESERVATION FOR THE TRANSIT.

CHOCOLATE BISCUITS

AUDIO RECORDER

MORE TOBACCO

53

THE CAMP'S **EXIT** IS LOCATED UNDERNEATH A BRIDGE WHICH CARRIES TRAFFIC TO AND FROM THE FERRY PORT.

(SEEN HERE FROM THE CAMP'S SOUTHERN PART WHICH GOT DEMOLISHED BY THE LOCAL AUTHORITIES A COUPLE OF WEEKS AGO.

BANKSY, THE BRITISH STREET ARTIST, CREATED A GRAFFITI DEPICTING STEVE JOBS, THE FOUNDER OF APPLE, CARRYING AN EARLY APPLE COMPUTER AND A BAG OF POSSESSIONS.

OTHER 'ARTISTS' HAVE REACTED AND ADDED WRITING...

Big Love from SCOTLAND

JOBS WAS BORN IN CALIFORNIA... HIS FATHER WAS A POLITICAL MIGRANT FROM THE SYRIAN CITY OF HOMS.

THE AFGHAN

AUTHOR'S NOTE:

On my last day in Calais I briefly met a tired and confused looking young Afghan. He did not want to be photographed and he didn't want his voice recorded.

The quotes on this spread are what I remember from what he told me...

THE FERRY PORT SEEN FROM FORT RISBAN.

UNTIL 1558 THE FORT, BACK THEN ALSO KNOWN AS FORT LANCASTER, WAS OCCUPIED BY THE ENGLISH.

← CONTRAIL OF AIRCRAFT CROSSING THE ENGLISH CHANNEL

① "I LIVED IN CROYDON ✱ FOR FIVE YEARS. BUT I GOT CAUGHT BY THE IMMIGRATION POLICE AND THEY PUT ME ON A FLIGHT TO KABUL.

✱ (BOROUGH IN SOUTH LONDON)

② "WHEN I WAS HERE IN CALAIS IN 2010 IT WASN'T EASY TO BOARD A TRUCK IN ORDER TO GET ON A FERRY. BUT IT WAS MUCH EASIER THAN IT IS NOW.

FLOOD LIGHTS

CCTV CAMERAS

RAZOR WIRE

Calais 5

ENGLAND

HADYA: "I WAS EXTREMELY WORRIED. JUST AFTER WISAM WENT TO SEA TWO OTHER MIGRANT BOATS SANK ON THEIR WAY TO ITALY... AROUND 800 PEOPLE DROWNED. I THOUGHT THAT WISAM WAS ON BOARD ONE OF THESE BOATS. I DIDN'T DARE TO TELL OUR CHILDREN AS THEY WERE ALREADY TRAUMATIZED BY PREVIOUS EVENTS AND I DIDN'T WANT TO WORRY THEM AS WELL." **WISAM:** "I TOOK TRAINS TO MILAN AND FROM THERE TO PARIS. ON MY JOURNEY FROM ITALY TO FRANCE I SPENT MORE THAN £600 ON TRAIN TICKETS! I THINK I SPENT TOO MUCH... I WAS LOST." **HADYA:** "I HAD SOME GOLD JEWELLERY THAT I SOLD. WE ALSO BORROWED MONEY TO PAY FOR WISAM'S JOURNEY." **WISAM:** "FROM PARIS I TRAVELLED ON TO CALAIS WHERE I WENT TO THE 'JUNGLE'. I DIDN'T LIKE THE PLACE... SO I WAS CAMPING OUT IN THE PORT AREA WHILST I WAS ATTEMPTING TO REACH GREAT BRITAIN. ONE DAY A COUPLE OF OTHER GUYS AND I PAID A SMUGGLER £4,000 EACH... IT WAS 'CHEAP' BACK THEN... NOW YOU WOULD HAVE TO PAY £7,000 TO £8,000 TO GET FROM CALAIS TO ENGLAND. THE GUY TOOK US TO A TRUCK AND SAID THAT THE TRUCK WAS SCHEDULED TO GO TO ENGLAND. HE OPENED THE DOORS AND LET US IN. IT WAS A REFRIGERATED TRAILER CARRYING BOXES OF CHOCOLATE. WE HID BEHIND THE BOXES AND THE SMUGGLER SHUT THE DOOR FROM THE OUTSIDE. BUT INSTEAD OF TAKING US TO ENGLAND THE TRUCK WENT TO BELGIUM. THERE WERE SEVERAL OTHER FAILED ATTEMPTS. BUT FINALLY ON THE 21ST DAY, THERE WERE THREE OF US, WE MANAGED TO GET IN A UK BOUND TRUCK. BUT THE DRIVER MUST HAVE SOMEHOW NOTICED US... HE OPENED THE DOOR AND DISCOVERED ONE OF US AND MADE HIM LEAVE THE TRAILER. BUT HE DIDN'T SEE US. AT THE FERRY PORT POLICE MEN ENTERED THE TRAILER. ONE OF THEM WAS ACTUALLY STANDING ON TOP OF THE BOX WE WERE HIDING IN... WE WERE PUTTING OUR HANDS AND KNEES UP, LIKE THAT, TO SUPPORT THE BOX. THEY DID NOT DISCOVER US. ABOUT ONE AND A HALF HOURS DRIVE AFTER WE HAD ARRIVED IN DOVER MY FRIEND FELT UNWELL. WE BANGED ON THE WALL NEXT TO THE DRIVER'S CABIN FOR ABOUT HALF AN HOUR UNTIL THE DRIVER STOPPED AND OPENED THE DOOR. MY FIRST VIEW OF ENGLAND WAS THE SURPRISED TRUCKER. I SAID 'THANK YOU' TO HIM (LAUGHS WHEN HE SAYS THIS). BUT HE WAS JUST GESTICULATING, SHOOING US AWAY SAYING 'GO, GO, GO!'. HE LEFT US IN THE MIDDLE OF NOWHERE... THERE WAS LOTS OF GREEN. I WAS SO HAPPY TO HAVE FINALLY ARRIVED IN ENGLAND. WE THEN TRIED TO STOP SOME CARS ON THE ROAD BUT NOBODY STOPPED. SO WE WENT TO A HOUSE FURTHER UP THE ROAD. I TOLD THE PEOPLE THERE 'POLICE, POLICE... I AM ARAB, I AM SYRIAN...!' I CROSSED MY WRISTS AS IF THEY WERE HANDCUFFED AND SAID: 'COME ON POLICE, POLICE...' ONE AND A HALF HOURS LATER THE POLICE CAME. THEY WERE VERY NICE AND TOOK US BACK TO DOVER WHERE THEY INTERVIEWED US. AFTERWARDS THEY DROVE US TO A HOSTEL IN LONDON, WHERE WE GOT ROOMS, A MEAL AND SOME MONEY. I THEN BOUGHT MYSELF A SIM CARD AND CALLED MY WIFE IN EGYPT."

RANEM (GIGGLING)

THIS WAS ON THE 18TH OF MAY 2015.

HADYA: "I WAS EXTREMELY HAPPY TO HEAR FROM HIM THAT HE ARRIVED SAFELY IN GREAT BRITAIN AND I GOT VERY EXCITED WITH THE PROSPECT OF JOINING HIM THERE SOON. OUR KIDS AND I ARRIVED IN BIRMINGHAM, VIA CAIRO AND ISTANBUL ON THE 22ND OF DECEMBER 2015. WE ARE VERY GRATEFUL TO THE RED CROSS WHO HELPED US OUT A LOT. THEY EVEN PAID FOR OUR TICKETS AS WE WERE OUT OF MONEY BY THEN. WHEN WE ARRIVED HERE THE COUNCIL PUT US UP IN A HOSTEL FOR SEVEN DAYS AND THEN THEY GAVE US THIS PLACE." **WISAM**: "BEFORE I WAS REUNITED WITH MY FAMILY I SPENT 14 DAYS IN LIVERPOOL AND IN PRESTON. I LIKED PRESTON A LOT... IT IS A GOOD PLACE... IT IS MUCH CALMER AND THE PEOPLE THERE WERE VERY GOOD." **HADYA**: "BUT I PREFER BIRMINGHAM BECAUSE MY WHOLE FAMILY LIVES HERE NOW." **WISAM**: "WE DON'T THINK THAT WE WILL GO BACK TO SYRIA ONE DAY... WE DON'T HAVE ANYTHING LEFT THERE NOW." **MOHAMAD**: "I AM NOT GOING TO GO BACK." **RANEM**: "I MISS MY AUNTS, THE SISTERS OF MY FATHER." (RANEM WAS 3 YEARS OLD WHEN SHE LEFT SYRIA). **MOHAMAD**: "I MISS OUR HOUSE IN SYRIA... I MISS PLAYING FOOTBALL AND TAG WITH MY OLD SCHOOL FRIENDS. BEFORE I CAME TO ENGLAND I DIDN'T REALLY KNOW ANYTHING ABOUT ENGLAND. I ONLY KNEW THAT MY FATHER WAS THERE AND THAT HE SAID THAT HE LIKED IT THERE AND THAT IT WAS A GOOD PLACE..." **WISAM**: "I CAN'T FIND WORK RIGHT NOW AS MY ENGLISH IS NOT GOOD ENOUGH." **MOHAMAD**: "I LIKE GOING TO SCHOOL IN BIRMINGHAM. I LEARN A LOT... I'VE GOT MANY FRIENDS. MY FAVOURITE SUBJECT IS PHYSICAL EDUCATION. I WANT TO BECOME THE CAPTAIN OF MY SCHOOL'S FOOTBALL TEAM."

① OUR FUTURE IN THE EMIRATES WOULD HAVE BEEN PRECARIOUS.

"ONCE MY CONTRACT WITH THE HOSPITAL HAD ENDED WE WOULD HAVE LOST THE RIGHT TO STAY IN THE COUNTRY. WE WOULD HAVE NEEDED A SPONSOR AND THERE IS NO SOCIAL SUPPORT SYSTEM FOR NON-LOCAL FAMILIES."

② THE EMIRATES WITH ALL ITS LUXURY IS A DREAM WORLD...

"LIVING THERE IS VERY EXPENSIVE! THE RENT, SCHOOLS, TRANSPORT... EVERYTHING. FORTUNATELY, AS I WAS A MEMBER OF THE MEDICAL STAFF, MY HUSBAND, MY CHILDREN AND I DIDN'T HAVE TO PAY FOR THE MEDICAL BILLS.

"HOWEVER MY INSURANCE DIDN'T COVER MY MOTHER WHO STAYED WITH US...

"SHE NEEDED PRIVATE HEALTH INSURANCE WHICH IS EXTREMELY EXPENSIVE OVER THERE.

③ I APPLIED FOR A UK-BUSINESS VISA AND BOOKED A FLIGHT TO GO TO LONDON.

"AFTER 14 DAYS I GOT MY PASSPORT WITH MY VISA IN IT. I WAS ABLE TO GET THE VISA BECAUSE I COULD PROVIDE STRONG BANK STATEMENTS... MY HUSBAND, UNFORTUNATELY, WASN'T ABLE TO ATTAIN A VISA.

"I CHOSE GOING TO THE UK BECAUSE I WENT TO LONDON IN 2008 TO ATTEND AN ANESTHESIA CONFERENCE AND I ENJOYED MY STAY A LOT.

④ "ALSO, IT MADE SENSE AS I LEARNT ENGLISH AS A SECOND LANGUAGE IN SYRIA AND DON'T THINK I'D MANAGE TO LEARN A THIRD LANGUAGE. I ALSO LIKED THE FACT THAT THERE IS A LARGE SYRIAN AND MUSLIM COMMUNITY IN THE UK.

⑤ "OF COURSE IT WAS VERY DIFFICULT FOR ME TO LEAVE MY FAMILY BEHIND. AT THE SAME TIME, THOUGH, I FELT A DOOR HAD OPENED AND WE THOUGHT THIS MIGHT BE A CHANCE WE WOULD NEVER GET AGAIN.

NOW IF THE HOME OFFICE GRANTS ME INDEFINITE LEAVE TO REMAIN AND IF I GET MY RESIDENCE CARD I CAN APPLY FOR FAMILY REUNION.

"MY HUSBAND, CHILDREN AND MOTHER ARE IN TURKEY NOW. THEY HAD TO LEAVE THE EMIRATES BECAUSE THEY WERE NOT ALLOWED

TO STAY THERE ANY LONGER AS THEIR VISA EXPIRED WHEN I LEFT FOR THE UK.

BACK THEN IT WAS STILL EASY FOR SYRIANS TO MOVE TO TURKEY WITHOUT A VISA.

THE MONEY I WAS ABLE TO SAVE IN THE EMIRATES PAYS FOR MY FAMILY'S LIVING EXPENSES IN ISTANBUL. BUT IT WON'T LAST FOR MUCH LONGER.

6 "I AM IN CONTACT WITH MY FAMILY VIA SKYPE.

I CAN'T IMAGINE A DAY WITHOUT SEEING THEM TWICE AT LEAST. I FIND IT VERY DIFFICULT TO TALK WITH MY CHILDREN. SOMETIMES IT IS NOT POSSIBLE AS THEY WOULD RATHER PLAY VIDEO GAMES, CAN YOU IMAGINE? WHEN THEY DO TALK WITH ME THEY START TO TELL ME HOW MUCH THEY MISS ME AND THEY EXPRESS THEIR FRUSTRATION ABOUT OUR SEPARATION UNTIL THEY START CRYING. I DON'T WANT THEM TO CRY ANYMORE SO I TRY NOT TO DIG TOO DEEP INTO THEIR EMOTIONS... I TRY NOT TO BE TOO AFFECTIONATE WITH THEM. OTHERWISE THEY WILL START ASKING ME AGAIN WHEN THEY WILL BE WITH ME NEXT... 'WHEN?! PLEASE GIVE ME A DATE.' I CAN'T GIVE THEM A DATE. MY DAUGHTER ACCUSED ME OF LYING TO HER. IN THE PAST I TOLD HER THAT, MAYBE, WE WILL BE REUNITED IN TWO OR THREE MONTHS... BUT WHEN THE TIME PASSED IT STILL HADN'T HAPPENED...

"I AM IN CONTACT WITH THE HOME OFFICE THROUGH MY MP RUPA HUQ... BUT THEY REPLIED THAT NO DECISION HAS BEEN MADE YET AND THAT THEY CAN'T GIVE ME ANY INFORMATION ABOUT WHEN THEY WILL BE ABLE TO MAKE A DECISION. I DON'T KNOW WHAT THEY ARE WAITING FOR... WHAT IS STOPPING THEM? MY CHILDREN NEED ME. MY DAUGHTER, I THINK, IS STARTING TO GET INTO PUBERTY... I TRY NOT TO THINK TOO MUCH ABOUT IT. I AM TRYING TO FOCUS ON IMPROVING MY ENGLISH SKILLS.

7 "I DON'T KNOW IF I'VE GOT THE RIGHT TO COMPLAIN. WHEN I HEAR OTHER PEOPLE'S STORIES I THINK MY STORY IS TRIVIAL. THERE ARE SO MANY PARENTS WHO LOST THEIR CHILDREN AND SO MANY CHILDREN BECAME ORPHANS.

SO I TRY NOT TO COMPLAIN, TO STAY QUIET AND TO BE PATIENT... I PRAY.

"MY CHILDREN SPEAK ENGLISH... AMERICAN ENGLISH! THEY WENT TO SCHOOLS WHERE THEY WERE TAUGHT BILINGUALLY. I WAS THINKING THAT MY CHILDREN HAVE NO IDENTITY... THEY WERE BORN IN THE EMIRATES AND DON'T SPEAK ARABIC WITH A DAMASCENE ACCENT... BUT NEITHER DO THEY SPEAK WITH AN EMIRATES ACCENT... AND NOW THEY ARE IN A TURKISH SCHOOL. LUCKILY THERE ARE MANY OTHER CHILDREN FROM SYRIA, IN FACT ALL THEIR FRIENDS ARE FROM DAMASCUS. THIS IS VERY COMFORTING FOR ME. MY CHILDREN KNOW NOW THAT THEY ARE SYRIAN. BEFORE, BEING SYRIAN, WAS JUST A VAGUE CONCEPT FOR THEM.

"I AM DOING VOLUNTARY WORK AT THE GREAT ORMOND STREET HOSPITAL ON A WARD, WHERE THE PATIENTS (CHILDREN) AND THEIR ACCOMPANYING MUMS ARE FROM OVERSEAS, MAINLY FROM ARABIC COUNTRIES. AT THE MOMENT I AM SUPPORTING A MUM WHOSE FOUR-MONTH-OLD CHILD IS RECEIVING CANCER TREATMENT. SO, IF THE MOTHER NEEDS TO TAKE A BREAK OR NEEDS TO HAVE A REST I LOOK AFTER HER BABY... I HOLD IT, FEED IT... CUDDLE IT.

"IDEALLY I WOULD LIKE TO WORK AS A DOCTOR IN THE UK... BUT I DON'T KNOW IF THIS WILL EVER BE POSSIBLE. THERE ARE MANY BARRIERS LIKE GETTING MY CERTIFICATE RECOGNIZED, THE LANGUAGE, THE TRAINING... I AM WORKING ON IT... I AM IN A BAD EMOTIONAL AND PHYSICAL SITUATION BUT I NEED TO BE STRONG."

73

GERMANY

'DREIFALTIGKEITSKIRCHE', SIMMOZHEIM ('TRINITY CHURCH')

7:20 A.M. NOUR AND SAAD LEAVE THE HOUSE AND WALK TO SCHOOL. (AUTHOR'S NOTE ①: I went to the same school when I was a little boy.)

IN SYRIA WE SAY NOUR, IN GERMANY I AM NORA. ✱

I AM IN 4TH GRADE AT THE ELEMENTARY SCHOOL HERE IN SIMMOZHEIM.

ENGLISH IS MY FAVORITE SUBJECT.

I AM ELEVEN YEARS OLD.

IT WAS MY BIRTHDAY TWO DAYS AGO!

I WANT TO BECOME A NURSE.

SAAD WANTS TO BECOME AN ENGINEER.

(LAUGHS!)

AUTHOR'S NOTE ②: My father told me:

"WHEN RABIE'S FAMILY ENTERED GERMANY AND CLAIMED ASYLUM AT THE BORDER, OFFICIALS PUT DOWN DATES IN EARLY JANUARY FOR ALL OF THE KIDS' BIRTHDAYS... ONLY THE PARENTS HAD PASSPORTS, WHICH NOTED THEIR ACTUAL BIRTHDAYS. AT THE TIME HUNDREDS OF THOUSANDS OF MIGRANTS WERE CROSSING THE BORDER... THERE PROBABLY WEREN'T ENOUGH TRANSLATORS TO PROPERLY REGISTER EVERYONE'S BIRTHDAY... THE OFFICIALS MUST HAVE BEEN TOTALLY OVERWHELMED. IT IS THE SAME WITH THE ERITREANS—SIX OUT OF EIGHT ERITREANS WE HAVE HERE IN SIMMOZHEIM WERE 'BORN' ON THE FIRST OF JANUARY."

✱ NOUR MEANS LIGHT IN ARABIC.

'GRUNDSCHULE' (ELEMENTARY SCHOOL)

72

KLETTER-WAND

<u>POSTSCRIPT:</u>

In February 2016, during a short stay in Switzerland, I had the chance to meet Nihad, the former member of <u>MSF</u>'s psychological team, who I met in Domiz two years previously. Niina Tanskanen, from MSF Zürich, joined me on this visit. She speaks Arabic.

In August 2015, Nihad and his wife Avin decided to leave the refugee camp with their little daughter Naz. The three of them started their exhausting and dangerous 21-day journey to Switzerland, via Turkey, Greece, Macedonia, Serbia, Hungary and Austria.

It was very nice to see Nihad again and to meet his small family. After a delicious Syrian lunch in their cozy flat, Nihad told me:

"I FELT VERY CLOSELY CONNECTED WITH MY PATIENTS IN DOMIZ AND I FOUND IT DIFFICULT TO LEAVE THEM. I OFTEN SUFFER FROM A BAD CONSCIENCE."

05.02.2016 WITTENBACH, CLOSE TO ST. GALLEN, SWITZERLAND. IN THE LIVING ROOM.

NIHAD IS WORRIED ABOUT HIS MOTHER. ✱ SHE IS STILL IN QAMISHLI.

CAT IN GERMAN → KATZE!

EINS, ZWEI, DREI... ← SHE CAN ALREADY COUNT TO TEN IN GERMAN.

AVIN, 23 YEARS OLD, STUDIED ECONOMICS IN ALEPPO.

NAZ, SHE HAD HER THIRD BIRTHDAY LAST WEEK.

↑ PRINCESS-DRESS (A BIRTHDAY PRESENT)

✱ Nihad's sick mother was granted a humanitarian visa to join them six months later, in the summer of 2016. Since then, she has lived with them.